# BLOOD PRESSURE TRACKER

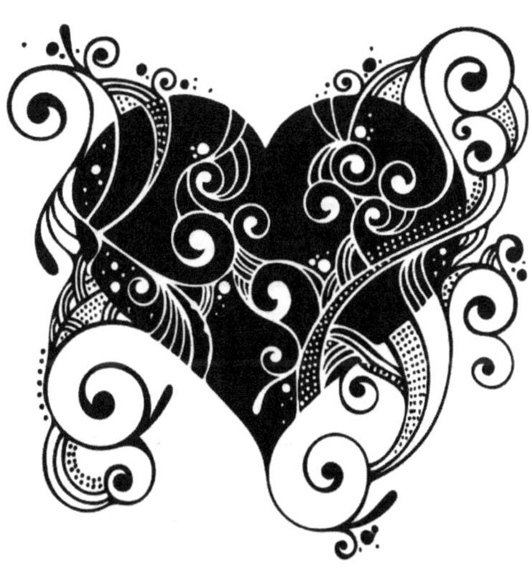

# Blood Pressure *Tracker*

| DATE | TIME | PRESSURE | PULSE | NOTES |
|------|------|----------|-------|-------|
|      |      |          |       |       |
|      |      |          |       |       |
|      |      |          |       |       |
|      |      |          |       |       |
|      |      |          |       |       |
|      |      |          |       |       |
|      |      |          |       |       |
|      |      |          |       |       |
|      |      |          |       |       |
|      |      |          |       |       |
|      |      |          |       |       |
|      |      |          |       |       |
|      |      |          |       |       |
|      |      |          |       |       |
|      |      |          |       |       |

# Blood Pressure *Tracker*

| DATE | TIME | PRESSURE | PULSE | NOTES |
|------|------|----------|-------|-------|
|      |      |          |       |       |
|      |      |          |       |       |
|      |      |          |       |       |
|      |      |          |       |       |
|      |      |          |       |       |
|      |      |          |       |       |
|      |      |          |       |       |
|      |      |          |       |       |
|      |      |          |       |       |
|      |      |          |       |       |
|      |      |          |       |       |
|      |      |          |       |       |
|      |      |          |       |       |
|      |      |          |       |       |
|      |      |          |       |       |

# Blood Pressure *Tracker* 

| DATE | TIME | PRESSURE | PULSE | NOTES |
|------|------|----------|-------|-------|
|      |      |          |       |       |
|      |      |          |       |       |
|      |      |          |       |       |
|      |      |          |       |       |
|      |      |          |       |       |
|      |      |          |       |       |
|      |      |          |       |       |
|      |      |          |       |       |
|      |      |          |       |       |
|      |      |          |       |       |
|      |      |          |       |       |
|      |      |          |       |       |
|      |      |          |       |       |
|      |      |          |       |       |
|      |      |          |       |       |

# Blood Pressure Tracker

| DATE | TIME | PRESSURE | PULSE | NOTES |
| --- | --- | --- | --- | --- |
|  |  |  |  |  |
|  |  |  |  |  |
|  |  |  |  |  |
|  |  |  |  |  |
|  |  |  |  |  |
|  |  |  |  |  |
|  |  |  |  |  |
|  |  |  |  |  |
|  |  |  |  |  |
|  |  |  |  |  |
|  |  |  |  |  |
|  |  |  |  |  |
|  |  |  |  |  |
|  |  |  |  |  |
|  |  |  |  |  |
|  |  |  |  |  |

# Blood Pressure *Tracker*

| DATE | TIME | PRESSURE | PULSE | NOTES |
|------|------|----------|-------|-------|
|  |  |  |  |  |
|  |  |  |  |  |
|  |  |  |  |  |
|  |  |  |  |  |
|  |  |  |  |  |
|  |  |  |  |  |
|  |  |  |  |  |
|  |  |  |  |  |
|  |  |  |  |  |
|  |  |  |  |  |
|  |  |  |  |  |
|  |  |  |  |  |
|  |  |  |  |  |
|  |  |  |  |  |
|  |  |  |  |  |
|  |  |  |  |  |

# Blood Pressure *Tracker*

| DATE | TIME | PRESSURE | PULSE | NOTES |
|------|------|----------|-------|-------|
|  |  |  |  |  |
|  |  |  |  |  |
|  |  |  |  |  |
|  |  |  |  |  |
|  |  |  |  |  |
|  |  |  |  |  |
|  |  |  |  |  |
|  |  |  |  |  |
|  |  |  |  |  |
|  |  |  |  |  |
|  |  |  |  |  |
|  |  |  |  |  |
|  |  |  |  |  |
|  |  |  |  |  |
|  |  |  |  |  |

# Blood Pressure *Tracker*

| DATE | TIME | PRESSURE | PULSE | NOTES |
|------|------|----------|-------|-------|
|  |  |  |  |  |
|  |  |  |  |  |
|  |  |  |  |  |
|  |  |  |  |  |
|  |  |  |  |  |
|  |  |  |  |  |
|  |  |  |  |  |
|  |  |  |  |  |
|  |  |  |  |  |
|  |  |  |  |  |
|  |  |  |  |  |
|  |  |  |  |  |
|  |  |  |  |  |
|  |  |  |  |  |
|  |  |  |  |  |

# Blood Pressure *Tracker*

| DATE | TIME | PRESSURE | PULSE | NOTES |
|------|------|----------|-------|-------|
|  |  |  |  |  |
|  |  |  |  |  |
|  |  |  |  |  |
|  |  |  |  |  |
|  |  |  |  |  |
|  |  |  |  |  |
|  |  |  |  |  |
|  |  |  |  |  |
|  |  |  |  |  |
|  |  |  |  |  |
|  |  |  |  |  |
|  |  |  |  |  |
|  |  |  |  |  |
|  |  |  |  |  |
|  |  |  |  |  |
|  |  |  |  |  |

# Blood Pressure Tracker

| DATE | TIME | PRESSURE | PULSE | NOTES |
|---|---|---|---|---|
|  |  |  |  |  |
|  |  |  |  |  |
|  |  |  |  |  |
|  |  |  |  |  |
|  |  |  |  |  |
|  |  |  |  |  |
|  |  |  |  |  |
|  |  |  |  |  |
|  |  |  |  |  |
|  |  |  |  |  |
|  |  |  |  |  |
|  |  |  |  |  |
|  |  |  |  |  |
|  |  |  |  |  |
|  |  |  |  |  |
|  |  |  |  |  |

# Blood Pressure *Tracker*

| DATE | TIME | PRESSURE | PULSE | NOTES |
|------|------|----------|-------|-------|
|      |      |          |       |       |
|      |      |          |       |       |
|      |      |          |       |       |
|      |      |          |       |       |
|      |      |          |       |       |
|      |      |          |       |       |
|      |      |          |       |       |
|      |      |          |       |       |
|      |      |          |       |       |
|      |      |          |       |       |
|      |      |          |       |       |
|      |      |          |       |       |
|      |      |          |       |       |
|      |      |          |       |       |
|      |      |          |       |       |
|      |      |          |       |       |

# Blood Pressure *Tracker*

| DATE | TIME | PRESSURE | PULSE | NOTES |
| --- | --- | --- | --- | --- |
| | | | | |
| | | | | |
| | | | | |
| | | | | |
| | | | | |
| | | | | |
| | | | | |
| | | | | |
| | | | | |
| | | | | |
| | | | | |
| | | | | |
| | | | | |
| | | | | |

# Blood Pressure Tracker

| DATE | TIME | PRESSURE | PULSE | NOTES |
|------|------|----------|-------|-------|
|  |  |  |  |  |
|  |  |  |  |  |
|  |  |  |  |  |
|  |  |  |  |  |
|  |  |  |  |  |
|  |  |  |  |  |
|  |  |  |  |  |
|  |  |  |  |  |
|  |  |  |  |  |
|  |  |  |  |  |
|  |  |  |  |  |
|  |  |  |  |  |
|  |  |  |  |  |
|  |  |  |  |  |
|  |  |  |  |  |

# Blood Pressure *Tracker*

| DATE | TIME | PRESSURE | PULSE | NOTES |
| --- | --- | --- | --- | --- |
|  |  |  |  |  |
|  |  |  |  |  |
|  |  |  |  |  |
|  |  |  |  |  |
|  |  |  |  |  |
|  |  |  |  |  |
|  |  |  |  |  |
|  |  |  |  |  |
|  |  |  |  |  |
|  |  |  |  |  |
|  |  |  |  |  |
|  |  |  |  |  |
|  |  |  |  |  |
|  |  |  |  |  |
|  |  |  |  |  |
|  |  |  |  |  |
|  |  |  |  |  |

# Blood Pressure *Tracker*

| DATE | TIME | PRESSURE | PULSE | NOTES |
| --- | --- | --- | --- | --- |
|  |  |  |  |  |
|  |  |  |  |  |
|  |  |  |  |  |
|  |  |  |  |  |
|  |  |  |  |  |
|  |  |  |  |  |
|  |  |  |  |  |
|  |  |  |  |  |
|  |  |  |  |  |
|  |  |  |  |  |
|  |  |  |  |  |
|  |  |  |  |  |
|  |  |  |  |  |
|  |  |  |  |  |
|  |  |  |  |  |

# Blood Pressure *Tracker*

| DATE | TIME | PRESSURE | PULSE | NOTES |
|------|------|----------|-------|-------|
|  |  |  |  |  |
|  |  |  |  |  |
|  |  |  |  |  |
|  |  |  |  |  |
|  |  |  |  |  |
|  |  |  |  |  |
|  |  |  |  |  |
|  |  |  |  |  |
|  |  |  |  |  |
|  |  |  |  |  |
|  |  |  |  |  |
|  |  |  |  |  |
|  |  |  |  |  |
|  |  |  |  |  |
|  |  |  |  |  |
|  |  |  |  |  |

# Blood Pressure Tracker

| DATE | TIME | PRESSURE | PULSE | NOTES |
| --- | --- | --- | --- | --- |
|  |  |  |  |  |
|  |  |  |  |  |
|  |  |  |  |  |
|  |  |  |  |  |
|  |  |  |  |  |
|  |  |  |  |  |
|  |  |  |  |  |
|  |  |  |  |  |
|  |  |  |  |  |
|  |  |  |  |  |
|  |  |  |  |  |
|  |  |  |  |  |
|  |  |  |  |  |
|  |  |  |  |  |
|  |  |  |  |  |
|  |  |  |  |  |

# Blood Pressure *Tracker*

| DATE | TIME | PRESSURE | PULSE | NOTES |
|------|------|----------|-------|-------|
|      |      |          |       |       |
|      |      |          |       |       |
|      |      |          |       |       |
|      |      |          |       |       |
|      |      |          |       |       |
|      |      |          |       |       |
|      |      |          |       |       |
|      |      |          |       |       |
|      |      |          |       |       |
|      |      |          |       |       |
|      |      |          |       |       |
|      |      |          |       |       |
|      |      |          |       |       |
|      |      |          |       |       |
|      |      |          |       |       |

# Blood Pressure Tracker

| DATE | TIME | PRESSURE | PULSE | NOTES |
|---|---|---|---|---|
| | | | | |
| | | | | |
| | | | | |
| | | | | |
| | | | | |
| | | | | |
| | | | | |
| | | | | |
| | | | | |
| | | | | |
| | | | | |
| | | | | |
| | | | | |
| | | | | |

# Blood Pressure *Tracker*

| DATE | TIME | PRESSURE | PULSE | NOTES |
|------|------|----------|-------|-------|
|      |      |          |       |       |
|      |      |          |       |       |
|      |      |          |       |       |
|      |      |          |       |       |
|      |      |          |       |       |
|      |      |          |       |       |
|      |      |          |       |       |
|      |      |          |       |       |
|      |      |          |       |       |
|      |      |          |       |       |
|      |      |          |       |       |
|      |      |          |       |       |
|      |      |          |       |       |
|      |      |          |       |       |
|      |      |          |       |       |

# Blood Pressure *Tracker*

| DATE | TIME | PRESSURE | PULSE | NOTES |
|------|------|----------|-------|-------|
|  |  |  |  |  |
|  |  |  |  |  |
|  |  |  |  |  |
|  |  |  |  |  |
|  |  |  |  |  |
|  |  |  |  |  |
|  |  |  |  |  |
|  |  |  |  |  |
|  |  |  |  |  |
|  |  |  |  |  |
|  |  |  |  |  |
|  |  |  |  |  |
|  |  |  |  |  |
|  |  |  |  |  |
|  |  |  |  |  |
|  |  |  |  |  |

# Blood Pressure *Tracker*

| DATE | TIME | PRESSURE | PULSE | NOTES |
|------|------|----------|-------|-------|
|      |      |          |       |       |
|      |      |          |       |       |
|      |      |          |       |       |
|      |      |          |       |       |
|      |      |          |       |       |
|      |      |          |       |       |
|      |      |          |       |       |
|      |      |          |       |       |
|      |      |          |       |       |
|      |      |          |       |       |
|      |      |          |       |       |
|      |      |          |       |       |
|      |      |          |       |       |
|      |      |          |       |       |
|      |      |          |       |       |
|      |      |          |       |       |

# Blood Pressure *Tracker*

| DATE | TIME | PRESSURE | PULSE | NOTES |
|------|------|----------|-------|-------|
|  |  |  |  |  |
|  |  |  |  |  |
|  |  |  |  |  |
|  |  |  |  |  |
|  |  |  |  |  |
|  |  |  |  |  |
|  |  |  |  |  |
|  |  |  |  |  |
|  |  |  |  |  |
|  |  |  |  |  |
|  |  |  |  |  |
|  |  |  |  |  |
|  |  |  |  |  |
|  |  |  |  |  |
|  |  |  |  |  |

# Blood Pressure Tracker

| DATE | TIME | PRESSURE | PULSE | NOTES |
|---|---|---|---|---|
|  |  |  |  |  |
|  |  |  |  |  |
|  |  |  |  |  |
|  |  |  |  |  |
|  |  |  |  |  |
|  |  |  |  |  |
|  |  |  |  |  |
|  |  |  |  |  |
|  |  |  |  |  |
|  |  |  |  |  |
|  |  |  |  |  |
|  |  |  |  |  |
|  |  |  |  |  |
|  |  |  |  |  |
|  |  |  |  |  |
|  |  |  |  |  |

# Blood Pressure Tracker

| DATE | TIME | PRESSURE | PULSE | NOTES |
|------|------|----------|-------|-------|
|  |  |  |  |  |
|  |  |  |  |  |
|  |  |  |  |  |
|  |  |  |  |  |
|  |  |  |  |  |
|  |  |  |  |  |
|  |  |  |  |  |
|  |  |  |  |  |
|  |  |  |  |  |
|  |  |  |  |  |
|  |  |  |  |  |
|  |  |  |  |  |
|  |  |  |  |  |
|  |  |  |  |  |

# Blood Pressure Tracker

| DATE | TIME | PRESSURE | PULSE | NOTES |
|------|------|----------|-------|-------|
|  |  |  |  |  |
|  |  |  |  |  |
|  |  |  |  |  |
|  |  |  |  |  |
|  |  |  |  |  |
|  |  |  |  |  |
|  |  |  |  |  |
|  |  |  |  |  |
|  |  |  |  |  |
|  |  |  |  |  |
|  |  |  |  |  |
|  |  |  |  |  |
|  |  |  |  |  |
|  |  |  |  |  |
|  |  |  |  |  |
|  |  |  |  |  |

# Blood Pressure *Tracker*

| DATE | TIME | PRESSURE | PULSE | NOTES |
|------|------|----------|-------|-------|
|      |      |          |       |       |
|      |      |          |       |       |
|      |      |          |       |       |
|      |      |          |       |       |
|      |      |          |       |       |
|      |      |          |       |       |
|      |      |          |       |       |
|      |      |          |       |       |
|      |      |          |       |       |
|      |      |          |       |       |
|      |      |          |       |       |
|      |      |          |       |       |
|      |      |          |       |       |
|      |      |          |       |       |
|      |      |          |       |       |

# Blood Pressure *Tracker*

| DATE | TIME | PRESSURE | PULSE | NOTES |
|------|------|----------|-------|-------|
|      |      |          |       |       |
|      |      |          |       |       |
|      |      |          |       |       |
|      |      |          |       |       |
|      |      |          |       |       |
|      |      |          |       |       |
|      |      |          |       |       |
|      |      |          |       |       |
|      |      |          |       |       |
|      |      |          |       |       |
|      |      |          |       |       |
|      |      |          |       |       |
|      |      |          |       |       |
|      |      |          |       |       |
|      |      |          |       |       |
|      |      |          |       |       |

# Blood Pressure Tracker

| DATE | TIME | PRESSURE | PULSE | NOTES |
| --- | --- | --- | --- | --- |
|  |  |  |  |  |
|  |  |  |  |  |
|  |  |  |  |  |
|  |  |  |  |  |
|  |  |  |  |  |
|  |  |  |  |  |
|  |  |  |  |  |
|  |  |  |  |  |
|  |  |  |  |  |
|  |  |  |  |  |
|  |  |  |  |  |
|  |  |  |  |  |
|  |  |  |  |  |
|  |  |  |  |  |
|  |  |  |  |  |

# Blood Pressure Tracker

| DATE | TIME | PRESSURE | PULSE | NOTES |
|------|------|----------|-------|-------|
|  |  |  |  |  |
|  |  |  |  |  |
|  |  |  |  |  |
|  |  |  |  |  |
|  |  |  |  |  |
|  |  |  |  |  |
|  |  |  |  |  |
|  |  |  |  |  |
|  |  |  |  |  |
|  |  |  |  |  |
|  |  |  |  |  |
|  |  |  |  |  |
|  |  |  |  |  |
|  |  |  |  |  |
|  |  |  |  |  |

# Blood Pressure *Tracker*

| DATE | TIME | PRESSURE | PULSE | NOTES |
| --- | --- | --- | --- | --- |
|  |  |  |  |  |
|  |  |  |  |  |
|  |  |  |  |  |
|  |  |  |  |  |
|  |  |  |  |  |
|  |  |  |  |  |
|  |  |  |  |  |
|  |  |  |  |  |
|  |  |  |  |  |
|  |  |  |  |  |
|  |  |  |  |  |
|  |  |  |  |  |
|  |  |  |  |  |
|  |  |  |  |  |
|  |  |  |  |  |

# Blood Pressure *Tracker*

| DATE | TIME | PRESSURE | PULSE | NOTES |
|---|---|---|---|---|
|  |  |  |  |  |
|  |  |  |  |  |
|  |  |  |  |  |
|  |  |  |  |  |
|  |  |  |  |  |
|  |  |  |  |  |
|  |  |  |  |  |
|  |  |  |  |  |
|  |  |  |  |  |
|  |  |  |  |  |
|  |  |  |  |  |
|  |  |  |  |  |
|  |  |  |  |  |
|  |  |  |  |  |
|  |  |  |  |  |

# Blood Pressure *Tracker*

| DATE | TIME | PRESSURE | PULSE | NOTES |
|---|---|---|---|---|
|  |  |  |  |  |
|  |  |  |  |  |
|  |  |  |  |  |
|  |  |  |  |  |
|  |  |  |  |  |
|  |  |  |  |  |
|  |  |  |  |  |
|  |  |  |  |  |
|  |  |  |  |  |
|  |  |  |  |  |
|  |  |  |  |  |
|  |  |  |  |  |
|  |  |  |  |  |
|  |  |  |  |  |
|  |  |  |  |  |
|  |  |  |  |  |

# Blood Pressure *Tracker*

| DATE | TIME | PRESSURE | PULSE | NOTES |
|------|------|----------|-------|-------|
|      |      |          |       |       |
|      |      |          |       |       |
|      |      |          |       |       |
|      |      |          |       |       |
|      |      |          |       |       |
|      |      |          |       |       |
|      |      |          |       |       |
|      |      |          |       |       |
|      |      |          |       |       |
|      |      |          |       |       |
|      |      |          |       |       |
|      |      |          |       |       |
|      |      |          |       |       |
|      |      |          |       |       |
|      |      |          |       |       |
|      |      |          |       |       |

# Blood Pressure Tracker

| DATE | TIME | PRESSURE | PULSE | NOTES |
|------|------|----------|-------|-------|
|  |  |  |  |  |
|  |  |  |  |  |
|  |  |  |  |  |
|  |  |  |  |  |
|  |  |  |  |  |
|  |  |  |  |  |
|  |  |  |  |  |
|  |  |  |  |  |
|  |  |  |  |  |
|  |  |  |  |  |
|  |  |  |  |  |
|  |  |  |  |  |
|  |  |  |  |  |
|  |  |  |  |  |

# Blood Pressure *Tracker*

| DATE | TIME | PRESSURE | PULSE | NOTES |
|------|------|----------|-------|-------|
|  |  |  |  |  |
|  |  |  |  |  |
|  |  |  |  |  |
|  |  |  |  |  |
|  |  |  |  |  |
|  |  |  |  |  |
|  |  |  |  |  |
|  |  |  |  |  |
|  |  |  |  |  |
|  |  |  |  |  |
|  |  |  |  |  |
|  |  |  |  |  |
|  |  |  |  |  |
|  |  |  |  |  |
|  |  |  |  |  |

# Blood Pressure *Tracker*

| DATE | TIME | PRESSURE | PULSE | NOTES |
| --- | --- | --- | --- | --- |
|  |  |  |  |  |
|  |  |  |  |  |
|  |  |  |  |  |
|  |  |  |  |  |
|  |  |  |  |  |
|  |  |  |  |  |
|  |  |  |  |  |
|  |  |  |  |  |
|  |  |  |  |  |
|  |  |  |  |  |
|  |  |  |  |  |
|  |  |  |  |  |
|  |  |  |  |  |
|  |  |  |  |  |
|  |  |  |  |  |
|  |  |  |  |  |
|  |  |  |  |  |

# Blood Pressure Tracker

| DATE | TIME | PRESSURE | PULSE | NOTES |
|------|------|----------|-------|-------|
|      |      |          |       |       |
|      |      |          |       |       |
|      |      |          |       |       |
|      |      |          |       |       |
|      |      |          |       |       |
|      |      |          |       |       |
|      |      |          |       |       |
|      |      |          |       |       |
|      |      |          |       |       |
|      |      |          |       |       |
|      |      |          |       |       |
|      |      |          |       |       |
|      |      |          |       |       |
|      |      |          |       |       |
|      |      |          |       |       |

# Blood Pressure Tracker

| DATE | TIME | PRESSURE | PULSE | NOTES |
|------|------|----------|-------|-------|
|      |      |          |       |       |
|      |      |          |       |       |
|      |      |          |       |       |
|      |      |          |       |       |
|      |      |          |       |       |
|      |      |          |       |       |
|      |      |          |       |       |
|      |      |          |       |       |
|      |      |          |       |       |
|      |      |          |       |       |
|      |      |          |       |       |
|      |      |          |       |       |
|      |      |          |       |       |
|      |      |          |       |       |
|      |      |          |       |       |
|      |      |          |       |       |

# Blood Pressure *Tracker*

| DATE | TIME | PRESSURE | PULSE | NOTES |
|------|------|----------|-------|-------|
|  |  |  |  |  |
|  |  |  |  |  |
|  |  |  |  |  |
|  |  |  |  |  |
|  |  |  |  |  |
|  |  |  |  |  |
|  |  |  |  |  |
|  |  |  |  |  |
|  |  |  |  |  |
|  |  |  |  |  |
|  |  |  |  |  |
|  |  |  |  |  |
|  |  |  |  |  |
|  |  |  |  |  |
|  |  |  |  |  |

# Blood Pressure *Tracker*

| DATE | TIME | PRESSURE | PULSE | NOTES |
|------|------|----------|-------|-------|
|  |  |  |  |  |
|  |  |  |  |  |
|  |  |  |  |  |
|  |  |  |  |  |
|  |  |  |  |  |
|  |  |  |  |  |
|  |  |  |  |  |
|  |  |  |  |  |
|  |  |  |  |  |
|  |  |  |  |  |
|  |  |  |  |  |
|  |  |  |  |  |
|  |  |  |  |  |
|  |  |  |  |  |
|  |  |  |  |  |
|  |  |  |  |  |

# Blood Pressure *Tracker*

| DATE | TIME | PRESSURE | PULSE | NOTES |
|------|------|----------|-------|-------|
|      |      |          |       |       |
|      |      |          |       |       |
|      |      |          |       |       |
|      |      |          |       |       |
|      |      |          |       |       |
|      |      |          |       |       |
|      |      |          |       |       |
|      |      |          |       |       |
|      |      |          |       |       |
|      |      |          |       |       |
|      |      |          |       |       |
|      |      |          |       |       |
|      |      |          |       |       |
|      |      |          |       |       |
|      |      |          |       |       |
|      |      |          |       |       |

# Blood Pressure *Tracker*

| DATE | TIME | PRESSURE | PULSE | NOTES |
|------|------|----------|-------|-------|
|  |  |  |  |  |
|  |  |  |  |  |
|  |  |  |  |  |
|  |  |  |  |  |
|  |  |  |  |  |
|  |  |  |  |  |
|  |  |  |  |  |
|  |  |  |  |  |
|  |  |  |  |  |
|  |  |  |  |  |
|  |  |  |  |  |
|  |  |  |  |  |
|  |  |  |  |  |
|  |  |  |  |  |
|  |  |  |  |  |
|  |  |  |  |  |

# Blood Pressure Tracker

| DATE | TIME | PRESSURE | PULSE | NOTES |
|------|------|----------|-------|-------|
|  |  |  |  |  |
|  |  |  |  |  |
|  |  |  |  |  |
|  |  |  |  |  |
|  |  |  |  |  |
|  |  |  |  |  |
|  |  |  |  |  |
|  |  |  |  |  |
|  |  |  |  |  |
|  |  |  |  |  |
|  |  |  |  |  |
|  |  |  |  |  |
|  |  |  |  |  |
|  |  |  |  |  |
|  |  |  |  |  |

# Blood Pressure Tracker

| DATE | TIME | PRESSURE | PULSE | NOTES |
|------|------|----------|-------|-------|
|  |  |  |  |  |
|  |  |  |  |  |
|  |  |  |  |  |
|  |  |  |  |  |
|  |  |  |  |  |
|  |  |  |  |  |
|  |  |  |  |  |
|  |  |  |  |  |
|  |  |  |  |  |
|  |  |  |  |  |
|  |  |  |  |  |
|  |  |  |  |  |
|  |  |  |  |  |
|  |  |  |  |  |
|  |  |  |  |  |

# Blood Pressure *Tracker*

| DATE | TIME | PRESSURE | PULSE | NOTES |
| --- | --- | --- | --- | --- |
|  |  |  |  |  |
|  |  |  |  |  |
|  |  |  |  |  |
|  |  |  |  |  |
|  |  |  |  |  |
|  |  |  |  |  |
|  |  |  |  |  |
|  |  |  |  |  |
|  |  |  |  |  |
|  |  |  |  |  |
|  |  |  |  |  |
|  |  |  |  |  |
|  |  |  |  |  |
|  |  |  |  |  |
|  |  |  |  |  |
|  |  |  |  |  |

# Blood Pressure *Tracker*

| DATE | TIME | PRESSURE | PULSE | NOTES |
| --- | --- | --- | --- | --- |
|  |  |  |  |  |
|  |  |  |  |  |
|  |  |  |  |  |
|  |  |  |  |  |
|  |  |  |  |  |
|  |  |  |  |  |
|  |  |  |  |  |
|  |  |  |  |  |
|  |  |  |  |  |
|  |  |  |  |  |
|  |  |  |  |  |
|  |  |  |  |  |
|  |  |  |  |  |
|  |  |  |  |  |
|  |  |  |  |  |
|  |  |  |  |  |

# Blood Pressure *Tracker*

| DATE | TIME | PRESSURE | PULSE | NOTES |
|------|------|----------|-------|-------|
|  |  |  |  |  |
|  |  |  |  |  |
|  |  |  |  |  |
|  |  |  |  |  |
|  |  |  |  |  |
|  |  |  |  |  |
|  |  |  |  |  |
|  |  |  |  |  |
|  |  |  |  |  |
|  |  |  |  |  |
|  |  |  |  |  |
|  |  |  |  |  |
|  |  |  |  |  |
|  |  |  |  |  |

# Blood Pressure Tracker

| DATE | TIME | PRESSURE | PULSE | NOTES |
|------|------|----------|-------|-------|
|      |      |          |       |       |
|      |      |          |       |       |
|      |      |          |       |       |
|      |      |          |       |       |
|      |      |          |       |       |
|      |      |          |       |       |
|      |      |          |       |       |
|      |      |          |       |       |
|      |      |          |       |       |
|      |      |          |       |       |
|      |      |          |       |       |
|      |      |          |       |       |
|      |      |          |       |       |
|      |      |          |       |       |

# Blood Pressure Tracker

| DATE | TIME | PRESSURE | PULSE | NOTES |
| --- | --- | --- | --- | --- |
|  |  |  |  |  |
|  |  |  |  |  |
|  |  |  |  |  |
|  |  |  |  |  |
|  |  |  |  |  |
|  |  |  |  |  |
|  |  |  |  |  |
|  |  |  |  |  |
|  |  |  |  |  |
|  |  |  |  |  |
|  |  |  |  |  |
|  |  |  |  |  |
|  |  |  |  |  |
|  |  |  |  |  |
|  |  |  |  |  |
|  |  |  |  |  |

# Blood Pressure *Tracker*

| DATE | TIME | PRESSURE | PULSE | NOTES |
|------|------|----------|-------|-------|
|  |  |  |  |  |
|  |  |  |  |  |
|  |  |  |  |  |
|  |  |  |  |  |
|  |  |  |  |  |
|  |  |  |  |  |
|  |  |  |  |  |
|  |  |  |  |  |
|  |  |  |  |  |
|  |  |  |  |  |
|  |  |  |  |  |
|  |  |  |  |  |
|  |  |  |  |  |
|  |  |  |  |  |
|  |  |  |  |  |

# Blood Pressure *Tracker*

| DATE | TIME | PRESSURE | PULSE | NOTES |
|---|---|---|---|---|
|  |  |  |  |  |
|  |  |  |  |  |
|  |  |  |  |  |
|  |  |  |  |  |
|  |  |  |  |  |
|  |  |  |  |  |
|  |  |  |  |  |
|  |  |  |  |  |
|  |  |  |  |  |
|  |  |  |  |  |
|  |  |  |  |  |
|  |  |  |  |  |
|  |  |  |  |  |
|  |  |  |  |  |
|  |  |  |  |  |
|  |  |  |  |  |

# Blood Pressure *Tracker*

| DATE | TIME | PRESSURE | PULSE | NOTES |
|------|------|----------|-------|-------|
|  |  |  |  |  |
|  |  |  |  |  |
|  |  |  |  |  |
|  |  |  |  |  |
|  |  |  |  |  |
|  |  |  |  |  |
|  |  |  |  |  |
|  |  |  |  |  |
|  |  |  |  |  |
|  |  |  |  |  |
|  |  |  |  |  |
|  |  |  |  |  |
|  |  |  |  |  |
|  |  |  |  |  |
|  |  |  |  |  |
|  |  |  |  |  |

# Blood Pressure Tracker

| DATE | TIME | PRESSURE | PULSE | NOTES |
|------|------|----------|-------|-------|
|  |  |  |  |  |
|  |  |  |  |  |
|  |  |  |  |  |
|  |  |  |  |  |
|  |  |  |  |  |
|  |  |  |  |  |
|  |  |  |  |  |
|  |  |  |  |  |
|  |  |  |  |  |
|  |  |  |  |  |
|  |  |  |  |  |
|  |  |  |  |  |
|  |  |  |  |  |
|  |  |  |  |  |
|  |  |  |  |  |
|  |  |  |  |  |

# Blood Pressure Tracker

| DATE | TIME | PRESSURE | PULSE | NOTES |
|---|---|---|---|---|
| | | | | |
| | | | | |
| | | | | |
| | | | | |
| | | | | |
| | | | | |
| | | | | |
| | | | | |
| | | | | |
| | | | | |
| | | | | |
| | | | | |
| | | | | |
| | | | | |
| | | | | |
| | | | | |

# Blood Pressure *Tracker*

| DATE | TIME | PRESSURE | PULSE | NOTES |
|------|------|----------|-------|-------|
|  |  |  |  |  |
|  |  |  |  |  |
|  |  |  |  |  |
|  |  |  |  |  |
|  |  |  |  |  |
|  |  |  |  |  |
|  |  |  |  |  |
|  |  |  |  |  |
|  |  |  |  |  |
|  |  |  |  |  |
|  |  |  |  |  |
|  |  |  |  |  |
|  |  |  |  |  |
|  |  |  |  |  |
|  |  |  |  |  |
|  |  |  |  |  |
|  |  |  |  |  |

# Blood Pressure *Tracker*

| DATE | TIME | PRESSURE | PULSE | NOTES |
| --- | --- | --- | --- | --- |
|  |  |  |  |  |
|  |  |  |  |  |
|  |  |  |  |  |
|  |  |  |  |  |
|  |  |  |  |  |
|  |  |  |  |  |
|  |  |  |  |  |
|  |  |  |  |  |
|  |  |  |  |  |
|  |  |  |  |  |
|  |  |  |  |  |
|  |  |  |  |  |
|  |  |  |  |  |
|  |  |  |  |  |
|  |  |  |  |  |

# Blood Pressure *Tracker*

| DATE | TIME | PRESSURE | PULSE | NOTES |
|------|------|----------|-------|-------|
|  |  |  |  |  |
|  |  |  |  |  |
|  |  |  |  |  |
|  |  |  |  |  |
|  |  |  |  |  |
|  |  |  |  |  |
|  |  |  |  |  |
|  |  |  |  |  |
|  |  |  |  |  |
|  |  |  |  |  |
|  |  |  |  |  |
|  |  |  |  |  |
|  |  |  |  |  |
|  |  |  |  |  |

# Blood Pressure *Tracker*

| DATE | TIME | PRESSURE | PULSE | NOTES |
|------|------|----------|-------|-------|
|      |      |          |       |       |
|      |      |          |       |       |
|      |      |          |       |       |
|      |      |          |       |       |
|      |      |          |       |       |
|      |      |          |       |       |
|      |      |          |       |       |
|      |      |          |       |       |
|      |      |          |       |       |
|      |      |          |       |       |
|      |      |          |       |       |
|      |      |          |       |       |
|      |      |          |       |       |
|      |      |          |       |       |
|      |      |          |       |       |

# Blood Pressure *Tracker*

| DATE | TIME | PRESSURE | PULSE | NOTES |
|------|------|----------|-------|-------|
|  |  |  |  |  |
|  |  |  |  |  |
|  |  |  |  |  |
|  |  |  |  |  |
|  |  |  |  |  |
|  |  |  |  |  |
|  |  |  |  |  |
|  |  |  |  |  |
|  |  |  |  |  |
|  |  |  |  |  |
|  |  |  |  |  |
|  |  |  |  |  |
|  |  |  |  |  |
|  |  |  |  |  |
|  |  |  |  |  |

# Blood Pressure Tracker

| DATE | TIME | PRESSURE | PULSE | NOTES |
|------|------|----------|-------|-------|
|  |  |  |  |  |
|  |  |  |  |  |
|  |  |  |  |  |
|  |  |  |  |  |
|  |  |  |  |  |
|  |  |  |  |  |
|  |  |  |  |  |
|  |  |  |  |  |
|  |  |  |  |  |
|  |  |  |  |  |
|  |  |  |  |  |
|  |  |  |  |  |
|  |  |  |  |  |
|  |  |  |  |  |
|  |  |  |  |  |

# Blood Pressure *Tracker*

| DATE | TIME | PRESSURE | PULSE | NOTES |
|------|------|----------|-------|-------|
|  |  |  |  |  |
|  |  |  |  |  |
|  |  |  |  |  |
|  |  |  |  |  |
|  |  |  |  |  |
|  |  |  |  |  |
|  |  |  |  |  |
|  |  |  |  |  |
|  |  |  |  |  |
|  |  |  |  |  |
|  |  |  |  |  |
|  |  |  |  |  |
|  |  |  |  |  |
|  |  |  |  |  |
|  |  |  |  |  |
|  |  |  |  |  |

# Blood Pressure *Tracker*

| DATE | TIME | PRESSURE | PULSE | NOTES |
|------|------|----------|-------|-------|
|      |      |          |       |       |
|      |      |          |       |       |
|      |      |          |       |       |
|      |      |          |       |       |
|      |      |          |       |       |
|      |      |          |       |       |
|      |      |          |       |       |
|      |      |          |       |       |
|      |      |          |       |       |
|      |      |          |       |       |
|      |      |          |       |       |
|      |      |          |       |       |
|      |      |          |       |       |
|      |      |          |       |       |
|      |      |          |       |       |
|      |      |          |       |       |

# Blood Pressure Tracker

| DATE | TIME | PRESSURE | PULSE | NOTES |
|------|------|----------|-------|-------|
|  |  |  |  |  |
|  |  |  |  |  |
|  |  |  |  |  |
|  |  |  |  |  |
|  |  |  |  |  |
|  |  |  |  |  |
|  |  |  |  |  |
|  |  |  |  |  |
|  |  |  |  |  |
|  |  |  |  |  |
|  |  |  |  |  |
|  |  |  |  |  |
|  |  |  |  |  |
|  |  |  |  |  |
|  |  |  |  |  |

# Blood Pressure Tracker

| DATE | TIME | PRESSURE | PULSE | NOTES |
| --- | --- | --- | --- | --- |
|  |  |  |  |  |
|  |  |  |  |  |
|  |  |  |  |  |
|  |  |  |  |  |
|  |  |  |  |  |
|  |  |  |  |  |
|  |  |  |  |  |
|  |  |  |  |  |
|  |  |  |  |  |
|  |  |  |  |  |
|  |  |  |  |  |
|  |  |  |  |  |
|  |  |  |  |  |
|  |  |  |  |  |
|  |  |  |  |  |
|  |  |  |  |  |

# Blood Pressure *Tracker*

| DATE | TIME | PRESSURE | PULSE | NOTES |
|------|------|----------|-------|-------|
|  |  |  |  |  |
|  |  |  |  |  |
|  |  |  |  |  |
|  |  |  |  |  |
|  |  |  |  |  |
|  |  |  |  |  |
|  |  |  |  |  |
|  |  |  |  |  |
|  |  |  |  |  |
|  |  |  |  |  |
|  |  |  |  |  |
|  |  |  |  |  |
|  |  |  |  |  |
|  |  |  |  |  |
|  |  |  |  |  |
|  |  |  |  |  |

# Blood Pressure Tracker

| DATE | TIME | PRESSURE | PULSE | NOTES |
|---|---|---|---|---|
|  |  |  |  |  |
|  |  |  |  |  |
|  |  |  |  |  |
|  |  |  |  |  |
|  |  |  |  |  |
|  |  |  |  |  |
|  |  |  |  |  |
|  |  |  |  |  |
|  |  |  |  |  |
|  |  |  |  |  |
|  |  |  |  |  |
|  |  |  |  |  |
|  |  |  |  |  |
|  |  |  |  |  |
|  |  |  |  |  |
|  |  |  |  |  |

# Blood Pressure *Tracker*

| DATE | TIME | PRESSURE | PULSE | NOTES |
|------|------|----------|-------|-------|
|      |      |          |       |       |
|      |      |          |       |       |
|      |      |          |       |       |
|      |      |          |       |       |
|      |      |          |       |       |
|      |      |          |       |       |
|      |      |          |       |       |
|      |      |          |       |       |
|      |      |          |       |       |
|      |      |          |       |       |
|      |      |          |       |       |
|      |      |          |       |       |
|      |      |          |       |       |
|      |      |          |       |       |
|      |      |          |       |       |
|      |      |          |       |       |

# Blood Pressure *Tracker*

| DATE | TIME | PRESSURE | PULSE | NOTES |
|------|------|----------|-------|-------|
|  |  |  |  |  |
|  |  |  |  |  |
|  |  |  |  |  |
|  |  |  |  |  |
|  |  |  |  |  |
|  |  |  |  |  |
|  |  |  |  |  |
|  |  |  |  |  |
|  |  |  |  |  |
|  |  |  |  |  |
|  |  |  |  |  |
|  |  |  |  |  |
|  |  |  |  |  |
|  |  |  |  |  |
|  |  |  |  |  |
|  |  |  |  |  |
|  |  |  |  |  |

# Blood Pressure Tracker

| DATE | TIME | PRESSURE | PULSE | NOTES |
|------|------|----------|-------|-------|
|  |  |  |  |  |
|  |  |  |  |  |
|  |  |  |  |  |
|  |  |  |  |  |
|  |  |  |  |  |
|  |  |  |  |  |
|  |  |  |  |  |
|  |  |  |  |  |
|  |  |  |  |  |
|  |  |  |  |  |
|  |  |  |  |  |
|  |  |  |  |  |
|  |  |  |  |  |
|  |  |  |  |  |
|  |  |  |  |  |

# Blood Pressure *Tracker*

| DATE | TIME | PRESSURE | PULSE | NOTES |
|---|---|---|---|---|
|  |  |  |  |  |
|  |  |  |  |  |
|  |  |  |  |  |
|  |  |  |  |  |
|  |  |  |  |  |
|  |  |  |  |  |
|  |  |  |  |  |
|  |  |  |  |  |
|  |  |  |  |  |
|  |  |  |  |  |
|  |  |  |  |  |
|  |  |  |  |  |
|  |  |  |  |  |
|  |  |  |  |  |
|  |  |  |  |  |

# Blood Pressure Tracker

| DATE | TIME | PRESSURE | PULSE | NOTES |
| --- | --- | --- | --- | --- |
|  |  |  |  |  |
|  |  |  |  |  |
|  |  |  |  |  |
|  |  |  |  |  |
|  |  |  |  |  |
|  |  |  |  |  |
|  |  |  |  |  |
|  |  |  |  |  |
|  |  |  |  |  |
|  |  |  |  |  |
|  |  |  |  |  |
|  |  |  |  |  |
|  |  |  |  |  |
|  |  |  |  |  |
|  |  |  |  |  |

# Blood Pressure Tracker

| DATE | TIME | PRESSURE | PULSE | NOTES |
| --- | --- | --- | --- | --- |
|  |  |  |  |  |
|  |  |  |  |  |
|  |  |  |  |  |
|  |  |  |  |  |
|  |  |  |  |  |
|  |  |  |  |  |
|  |  |  |  |  |
|  |  |  |  |  |
|  |  |  |  |  |
|  |  |  |  |  |
|  |  |  |  |  |
|  |  |  |  |  |
|  |  |  |  |  |
|  |  |  |  |  |
|  |  |  |  |  |
|  |  |  |  |  |

# Blood Pressure *Tracker*

| DATE | TIME | PRESSURE | PULSE | NOTES |
|---|---|---|---|---|
|  |  |  |  |  |
|  |  |  |  |  |
|  |  |  |  |  |
|  |  |  |  |  |
|  |  |  |  |  |
|  |  |  |  |  |
|  |  |  |  |  |
|  |  |  |  |  |
|  |  |  |  |  |
|  |  |  |  |  |
|  |  |  |  |  |
|  |  |  |  |  |
|  |  |  |  |  |
|  |  |  |  |  |
|  |  |  |  |  |

# Blood Pressure *Tracker*

| DATE | TIME | PRESSURE | PULSE | NOTES |
| --- | --- | --- | --- | --- |
|  |  |  |  |  |
|  |  |  |  |  |
|  |  |  |  |  |
|  |  |  |  |  |
|  |  |  |  |  |
|  |  |  |  |  |
|  |  |  |  |  |
|  |  |  |  |  |
|  |  |  |  |  |
|  |  |  |  |  |
|  |  |  |  |  |
|  |  |  |  |  |
|  |  |  |  |  |
|  |  |  |  |  |
|  |  |  |  |  |

# Blood Pressure *Tracker*

| DATE | TIME | PRESSURE | PULSE | NOTES |
| --- | --- | --- | --- | --- |
|  |  |  |  |  |
|  |  |  |  |  |
|  |  |  |  |  |
|  |  |  |  |  |
|  |  |  |  |  |
|  |  |  |  |  |
|  |  |  |  |  |
|  |  |  |  |  |
|  |  |  |  |  |
|  |  |  |  |  |
|  |  |  |  |  |
|  |  |  |  |  |
|  |  |  |  |  |
|  |  |  |  |  |
|  |  |  |  |  |
|  |  |  |  |  |

# Blood Pressure *Tracker*

| DATE | TIME | PRESSURE | PULSE | NOTES |
| --- | --- | --- | --- | --- |
|  |  |  |  |  |
|  |  |  |  |  |
|  |  |  |  |  |
|  |  |  |  |  |
|  |  |  |  |  |
|  |  |  |  |  |
|  |  |  |  |  |
|  |  |  |  |  |
|  |  |  |  |  |
|  |  |  |  |  |
|  |  |  |  |  |
|  |  |  |  |  |
|  |  |  |  |  |
|  |  |  |  |  |
|  |  |  |  |  |

# Blood Pressure *Tracker*

| DATE | TIME | PRESSURE | PULSE | NOTES |
|------|------|----------|-------|-------|
|      |      |          |       |       |
|      |      |          |       |       |
|      |      |          |       |       |
|      |      |          |       |       |
|      |      |          |       |       |
|      |      |          |       |       |
|      |      |          |       |       |
|      |      |          |       |       |
|      |      |          |       |       |
|      |      |          |       |       |
|      |      |          |       |       |
|      |      |          |       |       |
|      |      |          |       |       |
|      |      |          |       |       |
|      |      |          |       |       |
|      |      |          |       |       |

# Blood Pressure Tracker

| DATE | TIME | PRESSURE | PULSE | NOTES |
|------|------|----------|-------|-------|
|  |  |  |  |  |
|  |  |  |  |  |
|  |  |  |  |  |
|  |  |  |  |  |
|  |  |  |  |  |
|  |  |  |  |  |
|  |  |  |  |  |
|  |  |  |  |  |
|  |  |  |  |  |
|  |  |  |  |  |
|  |  |  |  |  |
|  |  |  |  |  |
|  |  |  |  |  |
|  |  |  |  |  |
|  |  |  |  |  |

# Blood Pressure *Tracker*

| DATE | TIME | PRESSURE | PULSE | NOTES |
| --- | --- | --- | --- | --- |
|  |  |  |  |  |
|  |  |  |  |  |
|  |  |  |  |  |
|  |  |  |  |  |
|  |  |  |  |  |
|  |  |  |  |  |
|  |  |  |  |  |
|  |  |  |  |  |
|  |  |  |  |  |
|  |  |  |  |  |
|  |  |  |  |  |
|  |  |  |  |  |
|  |  |  |  |  |
|  |  |  |  |  |
|  |  |  |  |  |

# Blood Pressure Tracker

| DATE | TIME | PRESSURE | PULSE | NOTES |
| --- | --- | --- | --- | --- |
|  |  |  |  |  |
|  |  |  |  |  |
|  |  |  |  |  |
|  |  |  |  |  |
|  |  |  |  |  |
|  |  |  |  |  |
|  |  |  |  |  |
|  |  |  |  |  |
|  |  |  |  |  |
|  |  |  |  |  |
|  |  |  |  |  |
|  |  |  |  |  |
|  |  |  |  |  |
|  |  |  |  |  |
|  |  |  |  |  |
|  |  |  |  |  |

# Blood Pressure *Tracker*

| DATE | TIME | PRESSURE | PULSE | NOTES |
|------|------|----------|-------|-------|
|  |  |  |  |  |
|  |  |  |  |  |
|  |  |  |  |  |
|  |  |  |  |  |
|  |  |  |  |  |
|  |  |  |  |  |
|  |  |  |  |  |
|  |  |  |  |  |
|  |  |  |  |  |
|  |  |  |  |  |
|  |  |  |  |  |
|  |  |  |  |  |
|  |  |  |  |  |
|  |  |  |  |  |
|  |  |  |  |  |
|  |  |  |  |  |

# Blood Pressure *Tracker*

| DATE | TIME | PRESSURE | PULSE | NOTES |
| --- | --- | --- | --- | --- |
|  |  |  |  |  |
|  |  |  |  |  |
|  |  |  |  |  |
|  |  |  |  |  |
|  |  |  |  |  |
|  |  |  |  |  |
|  |  |  |  |  |
|  |  |  |  |  |
|  |  |  |  |  |
|  |  |  |  |  |
|  |  |  |  |  |
|  |  |  |  |  |
|  |  |  |  |  |
|  |  |  |  |  |
|  |  |  |  |  |
|  |  |  |  |  |

# Blood Pressure *Tracker*

| DATE | TIME | PRESSURE | PULSE | NOTES |
|------|------|----------|-------|-------|
|      |      |          |       |       |
|      |      |          |       |       |
|      |      |          |       |       |
|      |      |          |       |       |
|      |      |          |       |       |
|      |      |          |       |       |
|      |      |          |       |       |
|      |      |          |       |       |
|      |      |          |       |       |
|      |      |          |       |       |
|      |      |          |       |       |
|      |      |          |       |       |
|      |      |          |       |       |
|      |      |          |       |       |
|      |      |          |       |       |

# Blood Pressure *Tracker*

| DATE | TIME | PRESSURE | PULSE | NOTES |
|------|------|----------|-------|-------|
|  |  |  |  |  |
|  |  |  |  |  |
|  |  |  |  |  |
|  |  |  |  |  |
|  |  |  |  |  |
|  |  |  |  |  |
|  |  |  |  |  |
|  |  |  |  |  |
|  |  |  |  |  |
|  |  |  |  |  |
|  |  |  |  |  |
|  |  |  |  |  |
|  |  |  |  |  |
|  |  |  |  |  |
|  |  |  |  |  |
|  |  |  |  |  |

# Blood Pressure *Tracker*

| DATE | TIME | PRESSURE | PULSE | NOTES |
|------|------|----------|-------|-------|
|  |  |  |  |  |
|  |  |  |  |  |
|  |  |  |  |  |
|  |  |  |  |  |
|  |  |  |  |  |
|  |  |  |  |  |
|  |  |  |  |  |
|  |  |  |  |  |
|  |  |  |  |  |
|  |  |  |  |  |
|  |  |  |  |  |
|  |  |  |  |  |
|  |  |  |  |  |
|  |  |  |  |  |
|  |  |  |  |  |
|  |  |  |  |  |

# Blood Pressure Tracker

| DATE | TIME | PRESSURE | PULSE | NOTES |
|------|------|----------|-------|-------|
|      |      |          |       |       |
|      |      |          |       |       |
|      |      |          |       |       |
|      |      |          |       |       |
|      |      |          |       |       |
|      |      |          |       |       |
|      |      |          |       |       |
|      |      |          |       |       |
|      |      |          |       |       |
|      |      |          |       |       |
|      |      |          |       |       |
|      |      |          |       |       |
|      |      |          |       |       |
|      |      |          |       |       |
|      |      |          |       |       |

# Blood Pressure Tracker

| DATE | TIME | PRESSURE | PULSE | NOTES |
| --- | --- | --- | --- | --- |
|  |  |  |  |  |
|  |  |  |  |  |
|  |  |  |  |  |
|  |  |  |  |  |
|  |  |  |  |  |
|  |  |  |  |  |
|  |  |  |  |  |
|  |  |  |  |  |
|  |  |  |  |  |
|  |  |  |  |  |
|  |  |  |  |  |
|  |  |  |  |  |
|  |  |  |  |  |
|  |  |  |  |  |
|  |  |  |  |  |
|  |  |  |  |  |
|  |  |  |  |  |

# Blood Pressure Tracker

| DATE | TIME | PRESSURE | PULSE | NOTES |
|------|------|----------|-------|-------|
|      |      |          |       |       |
|      |      |          |       |       |
|      |      |          |       |       |
|      |      |          |       |       |
|      |      |          |       |       |
|      |      |          |       |       |
|      |      |          |       |       |
|      |      |          |       |       |
|      |      |          |       |       |
|      |      |          |       |       |
|      |      |          |       |       |
|      |      |          |       |       |
|      |      |          |       |       |
|      |      |          |       |       |
|      |      |          |       |       |
|      |      |          |       |       |
|      |      |          |       |       |

# Blood Pressure *Tracker*

| DATE | TIME | PRESSURE | PULSE | NOTES |
| --- | --- | --- | --- | --- |
|  |  |  |  |  |
|  |  |  |  |  |
|  |  |  |  |  |
|  |  |  |  |  |
|  |  |  |  |  |
|  |  |  |  |  |
|  |  |  |  |  |
|  |  |  |  |  |
|  |  |  |  |  |
|  |  |  |  |  |
|  |  |  |  |  |
|  |  |  |  |  |
|  |  |  |  |  |
|  |  |  |  |  |
|  |  |  |  |  |

# Blood Pressure *Tracker*

| DATE | TIME | PRESSURE | PULSE | NOTES |
| --- | --- | --- | --- | --- |
|  |  |  |  |  |
|  |  |  |  |  |
|  |  |  |  |  |
|  |  |  |  |  |
|  |  |  |  |  |
|  |  |  |  |  |
|  |  |  |  |  |
|  |  |  |  |  |
|  |  |  |  |  |
|  |  |  |  |  |
|  |  |  |  |  |
|  |  |  |  |  |
|  |  |  |  |  |
|  |  |  |  |  |
|  |  |  |  |  |
|  |  |  |  |  |
|  |  |  |  |  |

# Blood Pressure *Tracker*

| DATE | TIME | PRESSURE | PULSE | NOTES |
|------|------|----------|-------|-------|
|  |  |  |  |  |
|  |  |  |  |  |
|  |  |  |  |  |
|  |  |  |  |  |
|  |  |  |  |  |
|  |  |  |  |  |
|  |  |  |  |  |
|  |  |  |  |  |
|  |  |  |  |  |
|  |  |  |  |  |
|  |  |  |  |  |
|  |  |  |  |  |
|  |  |  |  |  |
|  |  |  |  |  |
|  |  |  |  |  |
|  |  |  |  |  |

# Blood Pressure Tracker

| DATE | TIME | PRESSURE | PULSE | NOTES |
|------|------|----------|-------|-------|
|  |  |  |  |  |
|  |  |  |  |  |
|  |  |  |  |  |
|  |  |  |  |  |
|  |  |  |  |  |
|  |  |  |  |  |
|  |  |  |  |  |
|  |  |  |  |  |
|  |  |  |  |  |
|  |  |  |  |  |
|  |  |  |  |  |
|  |  |  |  |  |
|  |  |  |  |  |
|  |  |  |  |  |
|  |  |  |  |  |
|  |  |  |  |  |

# Blood Pressure Tracker

| DATE | TIME | PRESSURE | PULSE | NOTES |
|------|------|----------|-------|-------|
|  |  |  |  |  |
|  |  |  |  |  |
|  |  |  |  |  |
|  |  |  |  |  |
|  |  |  |  |  |
|  |  |  |  |  |
|  |  |  |  |  |
|  |  |  |  |  |
|  |  |  |  |  |
|  |  |  |  |  |
|  |  |  |  |  |
|  |  |  |  |  |
|  |  |  |  |  |
|  |  |  |  |  |
|  |  |  |  |  |

# Blood Pressure Tracker

| DATE | TIME | PRESSURE | PULSE | NOTES |
|---|---|---|---|---|
|  |  |  |  |  |
|  |  |  |  |  |
|  |  |  |  |  |
|  |  |  |  |  |
|  |  |  |  |  |
|  |  |  |  |  |
|  |  |  |  |  |
|  |  |  |  |  |
|  |  |  |  |  |
|  |  |  |  |  |
|  |  |  |  |  |
|  |  |  |  |  |
|  |  |  |  |  |
|  |  |  |  |  |
|  |  |  |  |  |

# Blood Pressure Tracker

| DATE | TIME | PRESSURE | PULSE | NOTES |
| --- | --- | --- | --- | --- |
|  |  |  |  |  |
|  |  |  |  |  |
|  |  |  |  |  |
|  |  |  |  |  |
|  |  |  |  |  |
|  |  |  |  |  |
|  |  |  |  |  |
|  |  |  |  |  |
|  |  |  |  |  |
|  |  |  |  |  |
|  |  |  |  |  |
|  |  |  |  |  |
|  |  |  |  |  |
|  |  |  |  |  |
|  |  |  |  |  |
|  |  |  |  |  |
|  |  |  |  |  |

# Blood Pressure *Tracker*

| DATE | TIME | PRESSURE | PULSE | NOTES |
| --- | --- | --- | --- | --- |
|  |  |  |  |  |
|  |  |  |  |  |
|  |  |  |  |  |
|  |  |  |  |  |
|  |  |  |  |  |
|  |  |  |  |  |
|  |  |  |  |  |
|  |  |  |  |  |
|  |  |  |  |  |
|  |  |  |  |  |
|  |  |  |  |  |
|  |  |  |  |  |
|  |  |  |  |  |
|  |  |  |  |  |
|  |  |  |  |  |
|  |  |  |  |  |

# Blood Pressure *Tracker*

| DATE | TIME | PRESSURE | PULSE | NOTES |
| --- | --- | --- | --- | --- |
|  |  |  |  |  |
|  |  |  |  |  |
|  |  |  |  |  |
|  |  |  |  |  |
|  |  |  |  |  |
|  |  |  |  |  |
|  |  |  |  |  |
|  |  |  |  |  |
|  |  |  |  |  |
|  |  |  |  |  |
|  |  |  |  |  |
|  |  |  |  |  |
|  |  |  |  |  |
|  |  |  |  |  |
|  |  |  |  |  |
|  |  |  |  |  |

# Blood Pressure Tracker

| DATE | TIME | PRESSURE | PULSE | NOTES |
|------|------|----------|-------|-------|
|      |      |          |       |       |
|      |      |          |       |       |
|      |      |          |       |       |
|      |      |          |       |       |
|      |      |          |       |       |
|      |      |          |       |       |
|      |      |          |       |       |
|      |      |          |       |       |
|      |      |          |       |       |
|      |      |          |       |       |
|      |      |          |       |       |
|      |      |          |       |       |
|      |      |          |       |       |
|      |      |          |       |       |

# Blood Pressure *Tracker*

| DATE | TIME | PRESSURE | PULSE | NOTES |
| --- | --- | --- | --- | --- |
|  |  |  |  |  |
|  |  |  |  |  |
|  |  |  |  |  |
|  |  |  |  |  |
|  |  |  |  |  |
|  |  |  |  |  |
|  |  |  |  |  |
|  |  |  |  |  |
|  |  |  |  |  |
|  |  |  |  |  |
|  |  |  |  |  |
|  |  |  |  |  |
|  |  |  |  |  |
|  |  |  |  |  |
|  |  |  |  |  |

# Blood Pressure *Tracker*

| DATE | TIME | PRESSURE | PULSE | NOTES |
|------|------|----------|-------|-------|
|      |      |          |       |       |
|      |      |          |       |       |
|      |      |          |       |       |
|      |      |          |       |       |
|      |      |          |       |       |
|      |      |          |       |       |
|      |      |          |       |       |
|      |      |          |       |       |
|      |      |          |       |       |
|      |      |          |       |       |
|      |      |          |       |       |
|      |      |          |       |       |
|      |      |          |       |       |
|      |      |          |       |       |
|      |      |          |       |       |

# Blood Pressure Tracker

| DATE | TIME | PRESSURE | PULSE | NOTES |
| --- | --- | --- | --- | --- |
|  |  |  |  |  |
|  |  |  |  |  |
|  |  |  |  |  |
|  |  |  |  |  |
|  |  |  |  |  |
|  |  |  |  |  |
|  |  |  |  |  |
|  |  |  |  |  |
|  |  |  |  |  |
|  |  |  |  |  |
|  |  |  |  |  |
|  |  |  |  |  |
|  |  |  |  |  |
|  |  |  |  |  |
|  |  |  |  |  |
|  |  |  |  |  |

# Blood Pressure Tracker

| DATE | TIME | PRESSURE | PULSE | NOTES |
|------|------|----------|-------|-------|
|      |      |          |       |       |
|      |      |          |       |       |
|      |      |          |       |       |
|      |      |          |       |       |
|      |      |          |       |       |
|      |      |          |       |       |
|      |      |          |       |       |
|      |      |          |       |       |
|      |      |          |       |       |
|      |      |          |       |       |
|      |      |          |       |       |
|      |      |          |       |       |
|      |      |          |       |       |
|      |      |          |       |       |
|      |      |          |       |       |

# Blood Pressure *Tracker*

| DATE | TIME | PRESSURE | PULSE | NOTES |
| --- | --- | --- | --- | --- |
|  |  |  |  |  |
|  |  |  |  |  |
|  |  |  |  |  |
|  |  |  |  |  |
|  |  |  |  |  |
|  |  |  |  |  |
|  |  |  |  |  |
|  |  |  |  |  |
|  |  |  |  |  |
|  |  |  |  |  |
|  |  |  |  |  |
|  |  |  |  |  |
|  |  |  |  |  |
|  |  |  |  |  |
|  |  |  |  |  |

# Blood Pressure Tracker

| DATE | TIME | PRESSURE | PULSE | NOTES |
| --- | --- | --- | --- | --- |
|  |  |  |  |  |
|  |  |  |  |  |
|  |  |  |  |  |
|  |  |  |  |  |
|  |  |  |  |  |
|  |  |  |  |  |
|  |  |  |  |  |
|  |  |  |  |  |
|  |  |  |  |  |
|  |  |  |  |  |
|  |  |  |  |  |
|  |  |  |  |  |
|  |  |  |  |  |
|  |  |  |  |  |
|  |  |  |  |  |
|  |  |  |  |  |

# Blood Pressure *Tracker*

| DATE | TIME | PRESSURE | PULSE | NOTES |
| --- | --- | --- | --- | --- |
| | | | | |
| | | | | |
| | | | | |
| | | | | |
| | | | | |
| | | | | |
| | | | | |
| | | | | |
| | | | | |
| | | | | |
| | | | | |
| | | | | |
| | | | | |
| | | | | |
| | | | | |

# Blood Pressure *Tracker*

| DATE | TIME | PRESSURE | PULSE | NOTES |
| --- | --- | --- | --- | --- |
|  |  |  |  |  |
|  |  |  |  |  |
|  |  |  |  |  |
|  |  |  |  |  |
|  |  |  |  |  |
|  |  |  |  |  |
|  |  |  |  |  |
|  |  |  |  |  |
|  |  |  |  |  |
|  |  |  |  |  |
|  |  |  |  |  |
|  |  |  |  |  |
|  |  |  |  |  |
|  |  |  |  |  |
|  |  |  |  |  |
|  |  |  |  |  |

# Blood Pressure *Tracker*

| DATE | TIME | PRESSURE | PULSE | NOTES |
|------|------|----------|-------|-------|
|  |  |  |  |  |
|  |  |  |  |  |
|  |  |  |  |  |
|  |  |  |  |  |
|  |  |  |  |  |
|  |  |  |  |  |
|  |  |  |  |  |
|  |  |  |  |  |
|  |  |  |  |  |
|  |  |  |  |  |
|  |  |  |  |  |
|  |  |  |  |  |
|  |  |  |  |  |
|  |  |  |  |  |
|  |  |  |  |  |

# Blood Pressure *Tracker*

| DATE | TIME | PRESSURE | PULSE | NOTES |
|------|------|----------|-------|-------|
|  |  |  |  |  |
|  |  |  |  |  |
|  |  |  |  |  |
|  |  |  |  |  |
|  |  |  |  |  |
|  |  |  |  |  |
|  |  |  |  |  |
|  |  |  |  |  |
|  |  |  |  |  |
|  |  |  |  |  |
|  |  |  |  |  |
|  |  |  |  |  |
|  |  |  |  |  |
|  |  |  |  |  |
|  |  |  |  |  |
|  |  |  |  |  |

# Blood Pressure Tracker

| DATE | TIME | PRESSURE | PULSE | NOTES |
|------|------|----------|-------|-------|
|  |  |  |  |  |
|  |  |  |  |  |
|  |  |  |  |  |
|  |  |  |  |  |
|  |  |  |  |  |
|  |  |  |  |  |
|  |  |  |  |  |
|  |  |  |  |  |
|  |  |  |  |  |
|  |  |  |  |  |
|  |  |  |  |  |
|  |  |  |  |  |
|  |  |  |  |  |
|  |  |  |  |  |
|  |  |  |  |  |
|  |  |  |  |  |

# Blood Pressure Tracker

| DATE | TIME | PRESSURE | PULSE | NOTES |
|------|------|----------|-------|-------|
|  |  |  |  |  |
|  |  |  |  |  |
|  |  |  |  |  |
|  |  |  |  |  |
|  |  |  |  |  |
|  |  |  |  |  |
|  |  |  |  |  |
|  |  |  |  |  |
|  |  |  |  |  |
|  |  |  |  |  |
|  |  |  |  |  |
|  |  |  |  |  |
|  |  |  |  |  |
|  |  |  |  |  |
|  |  |  |  |  |
|  |  |  |  |  |

# Blood Pressure *Tracker*

| DATE | TIME | PRESSURE | PULSE | NOTES |
|------|------|----------|-------|-------|
|  |  |  |  |  |
|  |  |  |  |  |
|  |  |  |  |  |
|  |  |  |  |  |
|  |  |  |  |  |
|  |  |  |  |  |
|  |  |  |  |  |
|  |  |  |  |  |
|  |  |  |  |  |
|  |  |  |  |  |
|  |  |  |  |  |
|  |  |  |  |  |
|  |  |  |  |  |
|  |  |  |  |  |
|  |  |  |  |  |

# Blood Pressure Tracker

| DATE | TIME | PRESSURE | PULSE | NOTES |
| --- | --- | --- | --- | --- |
|  |  |  |  |  |
|  |  |  |  |  |
|  |  |  |  |  |
|  |  |  |  |  |
|  |  |  |  |  |
|  |  |  |  |  |
|  |  |  |  |  |
|  |  |  |  |  |
|  |  |  |  |  |
|  |  |  |  |  |
|  |  |  |  |  |
|  |  |  |  |  |
|  |  |  |  |  |
|  |  |  |  |  |
|  |  |  |  |  |
|  |  |  |  |  |

# Blood Pressure Tracker

| DATE | TIME | PRESSURE | PULSE | NOTES |
|------|------|----------|-------|-------|
|  |  |  |  |  |
|  |  |  |  |  |
|  |  |  |  |  |
|  |  |  |  |  |
|  |  |  |  |  |
|  |  |  |  |  |
|  |  |  |  |  |
|  |  |  |  |  |
|  |  |  |  |  |
|  |  |  |  |  |
|  |  |  |  |  |
|  |  |  |  |  |
|  |  |  |  |  |
|  |  |  |  |  |
|  |  |  |  |  |
|  |  |  |  |  |

# Blood Pressure Tracker

| DATE | TIME | PRESSURE | PULSE | NOTES |
|------|------|----------|-------|-------|
|  |  |  |  |  |
|  |  |  |  |  |
|  |  |  |  |  |
|  |  |  |  |  |
|  |  |  |  |  |
|  |  |  |  |  |
|  |  |  |  |  |
|  |  |  |  |  |
|  |  |  |  |  |
|  |  |  |  |  |
|  |  |  |  |  |
|  |  |  |  |  |
|  |  |  |  |  |
|  |  |  |  |  |
|  |  |  |  |  |

# Blood Pressure *Tracker*

| DATE | TIME | PRESSURE | PULSE | NOTES |
|------|------|----------|-------|-------|
|      |      |          |       |       |
|      |      |          |       |       |
|      |      |          |       |       |
|      |      |          |       |       |
|      |      |          |       |       |
|      |      |          |       |       |
|      |      |          |       |       |
|      |      |          |       |       |
|      |      |          |       |       |
|      |      |          |       |       |
|      |      |          |       |       |
|      |      |          |       |       |
|      |      |          |       |       |
|      |      |          |       |       |
|      |      |          |       |       |
|      |      |          |       |       |

# Blood Pressure *Tracker*

| DATE | TIME | PRESSURE | PULSE | NOTES |
|---|---|---|---|---|
|  |  |  |  |  |
|  |  |  |  |  |
|  |  |  |  |  |
|  |  |  |  |  |
|  |  |  |  |  |
|  |  |  |  |  |
|  |  |  |  |  |
|  |  |  |  |  |
|  |  |  |  |  |
|  |  |  |  |  |
|  |  |  |  |  |
|  |  |  |  |  |
|  |  |  |  |  |
|  |  |  |  |  |
|  |  |  |  |  |

# Blood Pressure *Tracker*

| DATE | TIME | PRESSURE | PULSE | NOTES |
|------|------|----------|-------|-------|
|      |      |          |       |       |
|      |      |          |       |       |
|      |      |          |       |       |
|      |      |          |       |       |
|      |      |          |       |       |
|      |      |          |       |       |
|      |      |          |       |       |
|      |      |          |       |       |
|      |      |          |       |       |
|      |      |          |       |       |
|      |      |          |       |       |
|      |      |          |       |       |
|      |      |          |       |       |
|      |      |          |       |       |
|      |      |          |       |       |

# Blood Pressure *Tracker*

| DATE | TIME | PRESSURE | PULSE | NOTES |
| --- | --- | --- | --- | --- |
|  |  |  |  |  |
|  |  |  |  |  |
|  |  |  |  |  |
|  |  |  |  |  |
|  |  |  |  |  |
|  |  |  |  |  |
|  |  |  |  |  |
|  |  |  |  |  |
|  |  |  |  |  |
|  |  |  |  |  |
|  |  |  |  |  |
|  |  |  |  |  |
|  |  |  |  |  |
|  |  |  |  |  |
|  |  |  |  |  |
|  |  |  |  |  |

# Blood Pressure *Tracker*

| DATE | TIME | PRESSURE | PULSE | NOTES |
|------|------|----------|-------|-------|
|      |      |          |       |       |
|      |      |          |       |       |
|      |      |          |       |       |
|      |      |          |       |       |
|      |      |          |       |       |
|      |      |          |       |       |
|      |      |          |       |       |
|      |      |          |       |       |
|      |      |          |       |       |
|      |      |          |       |       |
|      |      |          |       |       |
|      |      |          |       |       |
|      |      |          |       |       |
|      |      |          |       |       |
|      |      |          |       |       |
|      |      |          |       |       |